CHAIR YOGA FOR SENIORS

STRETCHES FOR PAIN RELIEF AND JOINT HEALTH
THAT IMPROVE SENIORS' FLEXIBILITY TO HELP
PREVENT FALLS AND IMPROVE QUALITY OF LIFE

FIT FOREVER

CONTENTS

INTRODUCTION

Yoga is an ancient practice that has its roots in Eastern Asian tradition. It combines breathing, movement, and meditation to promote emotional, mental, and physical wellness. In the last few decades, yoga has become an increasingly popular form of exercise, particularly in the West. There are indeed many types and forms of yoga, but they are all designed to encourage overall health and wellness.

For many, traditional yoga can seem a bit overwhelming, especially for those of us who are no longer as steady on our feet as we once were or even for those of us who just feel better sitting. This is where chair yoga comes in!

Chair yoga offers all the benefits of traditional yoga but with the security of a chair to keep you firmly grounded. Like traditional yoga, chair yoga can help with pain and stress relief, and it can also assist with joint lubrication, balance, and the effects of arthritis.

This book has been specifically designed with seniors in mind who would like to begin or continue a yoga practice. It includes step-by-step guides for the various poses as well as variations depending on your comfort level. There are beginner, intermediate, and advanced chair poses that can be practiced as individual sequences or that can be combined to create a unique sequence that works for you.

Now that you've made the decision to add more movement to your daily routine, it is important that you consult with your doctor before you begin. Take the time to discuss your specific needs and how best to start your yoga practice. Not everyone will begin at the same level or progress in the same way. Once you've got the green light, remember to take it slow and do what feels right for you. Above all, have fun.

1

GETTING STARTED WITH CHAIR YOGA

As we age, our muscle strength declines affecting our legs, hips, and core. Chair yoga can help us to restore and maintain our spine health. Poor posture and weak spinal muscles can affect all parts of our bodies so having a regular chair yoga practice can help reverse or slow down some of the effects of aging on our bodies.

PSYCHOLOGICAL BENEFITS

Yoga connects the body to the mind and the mind to the spirit through the breath and helps us to be fully present in the moment and be aware. It can positively affect our mood as well as our cognitive function and can provide us with a sense of well-being and satisfaction.

Many seniors suffer from anxiety and worry, particularly about losing their independence or self-sufficiency. The focus on breathing and the breath in yoga can aid in soothing the mind and body and reducing the body's stress response. When practiced regularly, in a tranquil environment, it can alleviate stress and help bring peace and calm. We will explore the benefits of the breath in an upcoming chapter to better understand how breathing can impact the body and mood.

As with our physical bodies as we age, the structure and function of our brain change and decline. This can lead to impaired memory or reduced attention. Yoga can help stop the decline of brain function. In yoga, the brain has to focus and concentrate on performing the yoga poses or on meditating. This training of the brain to focus increases or improves attention, awareness, and memory (Hastings, 2017).

PHYSICAL BENEFITS

We have already established that physical activity, particularly for seniors, helps with mobility and strength as well as weight management and heart health. Yoga can improve balance, strength, and stability and can even slow down or reverse the loss of all of those. Just 20 minutes a day can improve your overall health and strength.

According to the Centers for Disease Control, falling is one of the main causes of injury and death among persons over 65 (Lehmkuhl, 2020). Being physically active and strengthening the muscles of your legs, hips, and core can go a long way in preventing falls and increasing your mobility. The more movement you can incorporate into your daily routine the better your balance will be. This means that you will be better able to perform your daily tasks. Staying physically active as you age can ensure that you maintain your independence.

As we age, our bones also become brittle, which means it is easier to break a bone if you fall. Doing yoga can help to strengthen your bones and delay or prevent the onset of osteoporosis. Yoga can, in fact, increase your bone density even as you get older.

Yoga can also increase your stamina and control joint inflammation and pain associated with many chronic conditions. This means that you can have the confidence to live and move independently.

The regular practice of yoga reduces your chance of having heart disease and of becoming a Type 2 diabetic. It also lowers your blood pressure and can alleviate aches and pains associated with aging. Importantly, it helps you to breathe better. Many people have difficulty breathing as they get older and a lack of oxygen to the cells can have detrimental effects on your body. Yoga teaches you how to focus on your breathing to maximize the flow of oxygen.

Yoga, or chair yoga in our case, can have a positive impact on our overall health—psychologically, emotionally, and physically. You can practice chair yoga anywhere, anytime in small groups or by yourself. You really don't need a lot to do it and the outcomes you gain by just doing 20 minutes a day are tremendous.

WHAT YOU NEED

As with any physical activity, it is always important to check with your doctor or healthcare professional before beginning. Chair yoga is a gentle form of exercise that does not have a lot of impact on the joints or muscles but it is still advisable to get the okay from your medical adviser.

For chair yoga, all you need is a non-cushioned chair with a straight back and no arms and, if possible, a set of two-pound hand weights and a yoga block. You should wear loose, comfortable clothing that is easy to move in and won't be restrictive. It is better to practice your yoga barefooted. If you're practicing on tiles or hardwood floors try to avoid socks because they may be slippery.

Find a space that works for you and that you will enjoy returning to on a daily basis. Make sure that the space you choose is big enough for your chair and you to fully extend your arms and legs. When choosing or creating your space, let it reflect your personality or what you want to feel in that space but don't let it be cluttered. Clutter will distract you from your practice. Remember the goal of your space should be to keep you calm, focused, and at peace.

Once you've found your space, the next step is to choose the time of day that works best for you. In the beginning, you may want to try doing your practice at different times and notice how you feel or if there are any distractions. Whatever time you choose, try to be consistent. It helps you to create a routine for your body and mind.

If you have never tried yoga before then it is probably best to start with the beginner poses and then work your way up as you get stronger and more confident. If you've been physically active you can opt for the intermediate poses but still check with your doctor first. Also, ensure that you are hydrated before and after your practice. Most importantly, relax and have fun.

2

BREATHING IN YOGA

Any yoga practice begins and ends with the breath. Breathing or *pranayama,* as it is called in yoga, is the quintessential feature of yoga. It is considered to be the *vital energy*. Awareness of your breath and matching your breathing to your movement is what defines yoga and makes it a whole-body experience as opposed to just an exercise.

When we become aware of our breath and our breathing, our mind becomes quieter, stiller. As a result, we become calmer and less agitated. Our breathing sends signals to our brain that, in turn, cause our bodies to react in certain ways. Breathing deeply and slowly tells our brain that everything is okay and that it is safe to relax and be at peace.

As we breathe deeply, the *vital energy* starts to push through our emotional and physical blockages and stresses. This movement of the *vital energy* throughout our body is what gives us the "feel good" sensation we experience at the end of our practice. In general, our heart beats more slowly when we exhale. Yoga uses breathing techniques to work with our body's natural responses to create that calming effect.

It is important to note though that *pranayama* is not rigorous breath control that results in discomfort or harm. It is also not an exercise; it is an awareness that can help to balance the physical, mental, and subtle bodies.

THE BREATH AND ITS BENEFITS

We've been breathing all our lives so we shouldn't need to be taught how to breathe, right? For the most part, this is true. Yoga is not about teaching you how to breathe properly; it's about helping you to become more aware of your breath and how it changes depending on what you're doing or how you're feeling. The notion of *pranayama* is to marry the breath to your activities, whether it's during your practice or your daily life. It is about paying attention and focusing on yourself—emotionally, mentally, and physically.

It is best to breathe in and out through your nose. Your nose is your body's natural air filter and can warm or cool the air as needed. The nose protects you against millions of foreign particles that circulate in the air. Moreover, breathing through your nose can reduce the rate of exertion during exercise or daily activities, which means that you will feel less tired during and after activity if you breathe through your nose. Furthermore, because the way we breathe sends signals to our brain, taking breaths through your nose reduces your nervous system's "fight or flight" response to situations.

Deep breathing and an awareness of your breath can lower your cortisol levels, the hormones responsible for stress. More importantly, it can help reduce your feelings of anxiety and depression. Focus on your breath can stabilize and even lower your blood pressure levels as well as strengthen your core. It can also counteract insomnia and sleeplessness. Overall, *pranayama* positively impacts your physical, emotional, and mental well-being.

BREATHING TECHNIQUES

Simple Breath

This technique is particularly beneficial for grounding and comfort and is the basis of many other breathing techniques.

1. Breathe in and out through your nose.
2. Begin to notice your breath without altering it.
3. Once you're comfortable, start to pay attention to the rhythm of your inhale and exhale.
4. Over time, begin to notice the space between your inhale and exhale as well as the pause between the two.
5. Continue as needed.

Yogic Breath

This technique helps to manage and ease anxiety and gives you that "feel good" sensation.

1. Begin with the simple breath technique.
2. When you're comfortable, begin to pay attention to the flow of air into the belly button towards the pubic bone as you breathe in and out and as the belly deflates as you breathe out.

3. Next, pay attention to how your rib cage expands as your belly button rises on your inhale and how your rib cage contracts and your belly deflates as you breathe out.
4. Allow yourself to become relaxed as your body embraces your breath.
5. Continue as needed until you are ready to complete your breathing practice.

Golden Thread Breath

If you suffer from insomnia or any kind of pain, this technique will provide the comfort and relief you need.

1. Start by establishing your yogic breath.
2. Once you are comfortable, begin to relax the muscles of your jaw and throat, and unclench your teeth. Create a small space between your teeth as well as your lips.
3. Keeping the breath gentle and steady, inhale through the nose and exhale through the tiny space between the lips.
4. Begin to focus on your exhale, and if possible, try to lengthen it slightly.
5. Continue this technique as desired, until you are ready to complete your practice.

Pranayama can benefit anyone and can be done anywhere. There is no special equipment or time frame. You simply take a few moments to bring awareness to your breath in any or all of your daily activities. Many times in yoga though, *pranayama* is part of a broader meditation practice. We will briefly explore meditation in the next chapter before moving on to the chair yoga poses.

3

MEDITATION

Meditation has been practiced by many different cultures worldwide for centuries. In its literal sense, meditation means to reflect upon or contemplate. In yoga, meditation relates to the awareness of the interconnectedness of all living things. It is more than simply concentration; it is a widening of your state of awareness. The first step in meditation is stilling the mind. This in turn relaxes your nervous system and allows you to focus and become aware of things around you.

Chair yoga is great because the poses in this form of yoga can be meditative in and of themselves. *Pranayama* and the yoga poses combined help to prepare your body for meditation by encouraging us to focus on our posture and our breathing. Additionally, like chair yoga itself, meditation can be practiced anywhere, at any time.

IMPORTANCE AND BENEFITS OF MEDITATION

We often rush through our days and our routines, not paying attention to the steps and details that led us through these moments. We tend to be disconnected from our present, many times because we are focused on what is supposed to happen next or worrying about what came before.

Meditation helps to center and ground us and make us more mindful, not only of our surroundings but of our actions and thoughts. It can create feelings of peace and ease and can help to release your body of unwanted tension. Through meditation and the expansion of your awareness, you give your active mind a chance to rest and release the constant thoughts and stressors.

In effect, a regular meditation practice can act as a form of stress management and aid in increasing your emotional well-being. It may also aid in managing your symptoms of anxiety, depression, sleeplessness, and pain. Meditation also improves your memory and can boost your immunity.

Combining *pranayama* with your meditation practice is beneficial to your overall health and wellness. It will leave you feeling alert and refreshed. Meditation is a great way to begin or end your day or to help you deal with any difficulties that may arise during the course of your day.

PRACTICING CHAIR MEDITATION

Before you embark on a meditation practice, it is important for you to remember to be patient and kind to yourself. Meditation takes time so start slowly, for short periods of time. Don't expect to be able to meditate for 30 minutes on your first try. It is a practice because you have to train your mind and body to relax and be receptive.

Like your yoga practice, you also need to set a schedule for your meditation practice. Again, find the time of day that works best for you and has the least amount of disruptions or interruptions. It may be easiest to practice your meditation at the end of your yoga chair practice. Create a space that is comfortable and welcoming and free from clutter.

Most importantly, be comfortable. If you are fidgeting or in any distress, you will not gain the benefits of your practice. There is no one posture for meditation. Select the way that you can sustain for the length of your practice and again, choose clothing that is loose and easy to move in.

Chair Meditation

1. Sit up tall in your chair and place your feet flat on the floor, hip-distance apart. Slouching will constrict your breathing.
2. Ground down through your sitz bones (bottom part of your pelvis) and relax your shoulders back and down, away from your ears.
3. If it feels comfortable, close your eyes or gently lower and soften your gaze. Rest your hands on your thighs with your palms facing up. This gesture creates openness and receptivity.
4. Begin to notice your breath and perhaps practice one of the breathing techniques.
5. To come out of your meditation, begin to return to your normal breathing, then gently open your eyes. Give yourself a moment to assimilate the sensations.

BEGINNER POSES

If you're just getting started with a physical fitness routine or you're new to yoga then this is a great place to start. The yoga poses in this section are meant to provide you with a firm foundation. They are the poses you can use as you build your practice and you will be able to add more to them as you move along.

The poses highlighted here can be done in sequence to provide you with a 20-minute practice. If you include *pranayama* and meditation at the end of the sequence you will have about a 30-minute practice. Most importantly, take your time and enjoy each moment of your practice.

MOUNTAIN POSE

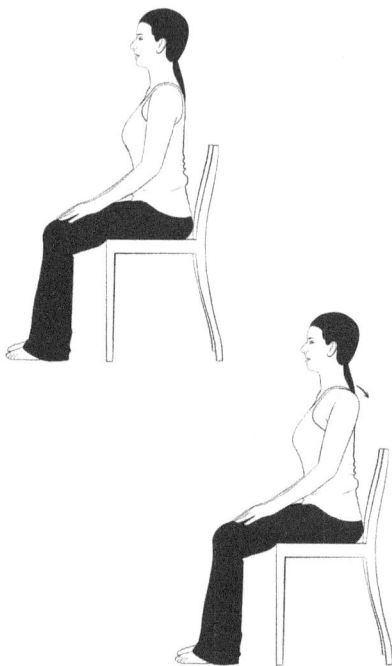

This is a great pose to begin your practice. It engages your core muscles as you sit up tall and helps you focus on your breath and check in with your posture. You can return to this pose after each pose in the sequence.

To begin:

1. Take a deep inhale and sit up tall in your chair, extending your spine.
2. Keep your feet flat on the floor with your knees hip-width apart and your toes pointing forward. Rest your hands, palms facing up, gently on your thighs.
3. Take another deep breath in and as you exhale, gently roll your shoulders back and away from your ears.
4. Engage your core as you become heavy on your sitting bones and lengthen through your spine. Keep your feet firmly pressed into the ground.

SIDE NECK STRETCHES

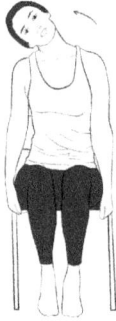

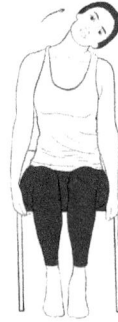

These stretches are a great way to reduce tension in the neck and shoulders and help you to relax your jaw and facial muscles.

1. Begin in Mountain pose.
2. Sit up tall as you inhale.

3. As you exhale, slowly drop your right ear to your right shoulder. Notice if your shoulders are tense and reaching towards your ear. Try to relax your shoulders and roll them back and down.
4. Inhale and lift your head back up to a neutral position.
5. Now, exhale again and drop your left ear to your left shoulder. Again, observe your shoulders and try to keep them relaxed and down, away from the ears.
6. Inhale and return your head to its neutral position.
7. Try to do this pose at least 3 times on each side. You can do more if it feels good and you feel that your body needs it.

SHOULDER ROLLS

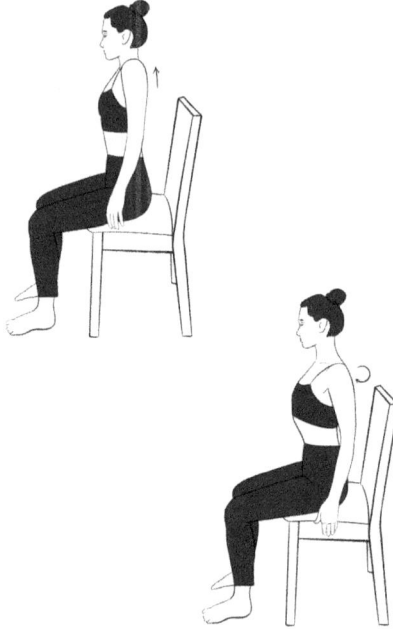

Shoulder rolls help to open up the shoulders and improve mobility in the shoulder joints. This ensures that you can easily and confidently complete daily tasks.

1. Begin by sitting in Mountain pose.
2. Inhale and lift your shoulders up, then back. As you exhale, bring your shoulders down and around back to your starting position. You should make a full circle with your shoulders with each cycle of breath.
3. Try to keep the movement of your shoulders smooth and continuous.
4. After five circles like this, reverse the movement bringing your shoulders up and forward as you inhale and down and around as you return to the start. This direction may feel a bit strange but that's how it should be. Complete five circles in this direction.

VOLCANO ARMS

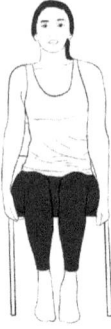

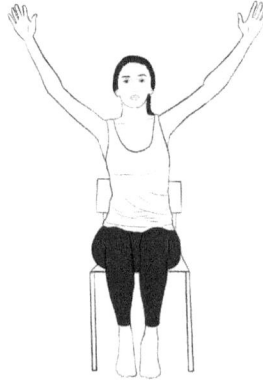

This pose gently stretches your shoulders, arms, and chest and can help improve your mobility in the shoulder joints.

1. Start in Mountain pose.
2. As you inhale, slowly begin to lift both arms above your head in the shape of a V. Notice if

your shoulders are lifting up towards your ears and try to relax your shoulders down.

3. As you exhale, lower your arms to the starting position.
4. Repeat this pose at least 3 more times and try to match your breathing to your movements. If it feels uncomfortable to lift your arms all the way up, just go as far as feels good and doesn't cause any discomfort.

SEATED ONE-LEGGED MOUNTAIN

This pose engages your core muscles, which are critical for sitting, standing, walking, and movement in general. It also helps to tone and strengthen your quadriceps.

1. Begin in Mountain pose, sitting up tall with your shoulders relaxed away from your ears and your feet firmly on the floor with your legs at right angles.
2. Inhale and slowly lift your right knee up and then lower it. Only lift your knee as high as feels good to you. You should not feel any pain or discomfort. Lower your foot as you exhale.
3. Repeat this ten times with each leg, then return to the Mountain pose and observe your breath.

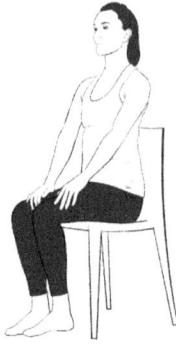

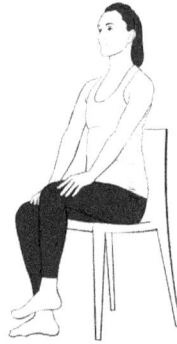

KNEE SWINGS

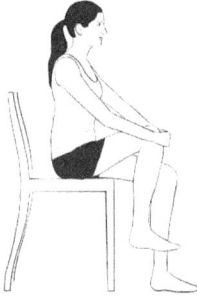

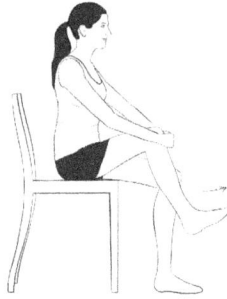

Knee swings are a good way to strengthen the muscles around your knees. They also help to increase the range of motion and mobility in your knees. Strong knee muscles and joints can protect you from knee injuries as you age.

1. Begin in Mountain pose with your belly button pulled in and your shoulders relaxed away from your ears.

2. If you can, clasp your hand under your right knee and begin to kick your right leg back and forth. If reaching under your knee is difficult, you can sit back in your chair and kick your right leg back and forth.

3. Repeat these steps for your left leg. Remember, only lift your leg as high as feels comfortable and go at a pace that is sustainable for you. Also, make sure you note your breath.

4. Try to do at least 10 swings on each side.

LEG LIFTS WITH POINT AND FLEX

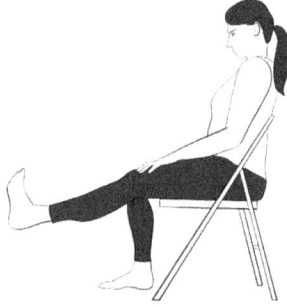

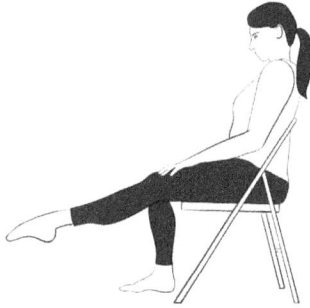

Leg lifts are good for toning your quadriceps and engaging your core. Pointing and flexing your feet help to stretch the muscles in your shin and calf and increases mobility in the foot.

1. Start by sitting up tall in your chair with your feet firmly touching the ground and your hands resting anywhere that is comfortable.
2. As you breathe in, extend your right leg out in front of you. Only go as high or as far as feels good for you. With your leg extended, point and flex your right foot a few times. This can be done quickly or slowly depending on how you feel.
3. On an exhale, slowly lower your right foot.
4. Repeat the movement with your left leg and foot and try to do at least five on each side. As you get stronger and more confident you can increase the number of lifts.

FULL BODY STRETCH

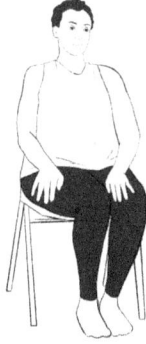

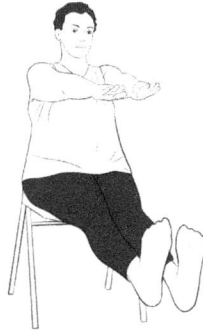

This pose engages all the muscles in your body and helps to strengthen them. It is also a great way to end your practice.

1. Begin in Mountain pose with your knees hip-width apart and your core engaged.

2. As you inhale, slowly and gently lift your arms and legs up at the same time. Try not to slouch as you do this. Only lift as far as you can.

3. On an exhale, return to the Mountain pose. Repeat this movement at least three times.

4. When you return to the Mountain pose after your last stretch, take a few minutes to relax and observe your breath and the sensations in your body.

5

INTERMEDIATE POSES

As you get stronger or if you are physically active then you may consider trying these poses. You can add them to the Beginner poses for a longer, more fluid practice or you can do them on their own. No matter what you decide, you will benefit from this practice. For these poses, you can add a set of two-pound weights. As always, check with your doctor before you begin, be sure to stay hydrated, and have fun.

SHOULDER ROLLS WITH HANDS

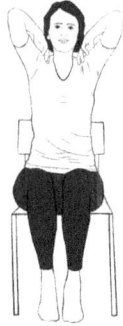

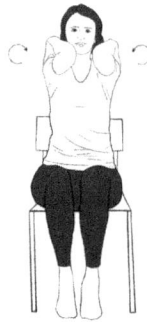

This movement is great for warming up your upper back and shoulders and releasing any tension. It also increases mobility in the shoulder joints.

1. Begin in Mountain pose and place your fingertips on your shoulders.

2. Begin to make circles with your shoulders, using your elbows to guide you. Go as slow or as fast as feels comfortable and be sure to notice your breath as you do your circles.
3. After five complete circles in one direction, reverse your circles and do five more.

WARRIOR II ARMS WITH FISTS

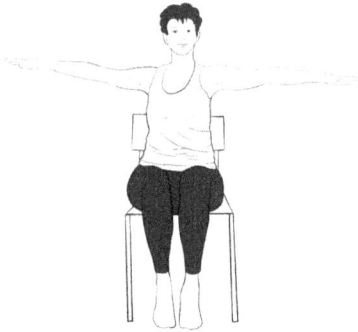

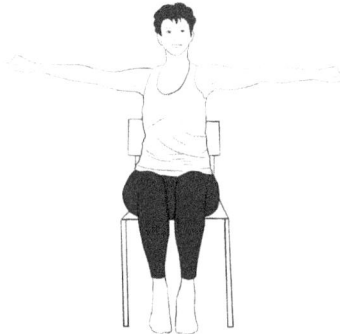

This pose engages the muscles of your upper arms and shoulders and strengthens your hands and fingers. It is especially beneficial to those suffering from carpal tunnel syndrome.

1. Start in Mountain pose, making sure that your feet are firmly planted on the ground and that you are sitting up straight. Remember, slouching will diminish your breathing and make the pose more difficult.
2. Slowly extend both arms up and out to your sides until they are shoulder level. Don't worry if you can't quite reach there yet, just go as far as you can.
3. Keeping your arms lifted, inhale and squeeze your fingers into tight fists. As you exhale, stretch the fingers as wide as you can, exaggerating the movement. Lower the arms.
4. Repeat this movement at least eight more times.

SEATED SIDE TWIST

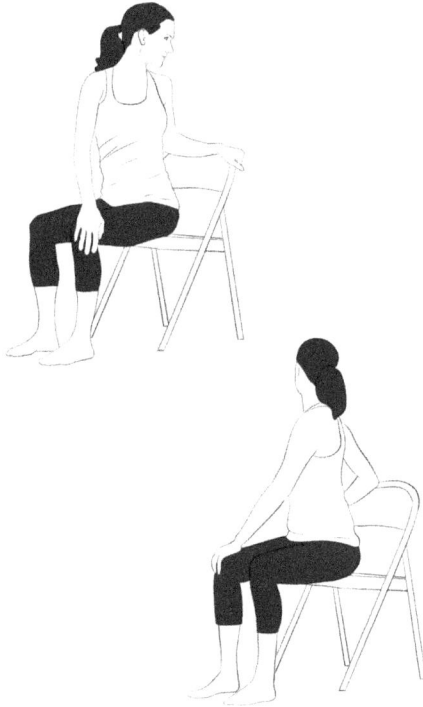

The movements involved in this pose help to tone your waistline while engaging your core. It also increases flexibility in your spine.

1. Again, begin in Mountain pose keeping a nice straight back with your shoulders down and away from your ears.
2. Inhale and gently twist to the right, placing your left hand on your right knee. Turn your head to look to your right, gazing toward or over your right shoulder.
3. Inhale during your twist and try to sit up taller. On your exhale, return to the Mountain pose.
4. Inhale again and gently twist to your left, placing your right hand on your left knee. Notice your breathing as you sit up tall. Exhale and return to the Mountain pose.
5. Repeat this pose five times on each side.

SEATED FORWARD FOLD

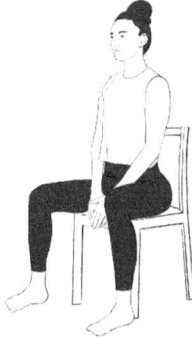

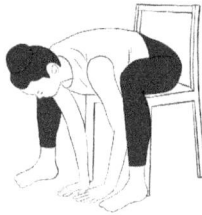

This posture increases the mobility in your back while strengthening the muscles of your lower back. It also provides an incredible stretch for your back, neck, and shoulders.

1. Begin by sitting up tall in your chair with your feet facing forward and firmly on the ground and your palms resting on your thighs.
2. Inhale, and with your back straight, begin to lean forward from your hips as if you're peering into a pond. Only go as far as you can while keeping your back straight.
3. As you exhale, engage the muscles of your core, and using your hands for support, lift back up to a seated position.
4. Repeat this movement at least five times. Your movements may be big or small depending on the flexibility of your spine and the mobility of your hips. Don't worry about it. As you strengthen your muscles, you will increase your flexibility.

BACKBEND

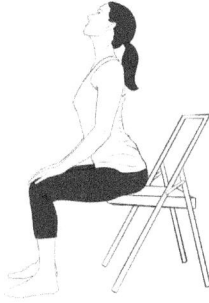

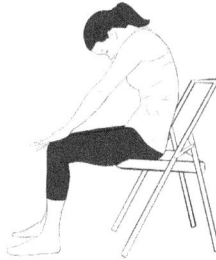

This posture is great for warming up the upper and lower back and is a counterpose to the seated forward fold. It also helps with your posture.

1. Begin in Mountain pose with your palms resting on the tops of your thighs.

2. As you inhale, slowly lift your chin, open your chest and shoulders, and slightly arch your back, looking up at the ceiling.

3. On your exhale, lower your chin to your chest, drop your head, and round your shoulders looking down at the floor.

4. Try to get the movements to flow with your breath. Do this movement at least five times.

SEATED TO CHAIR POSE

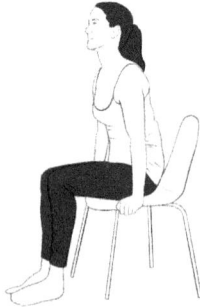

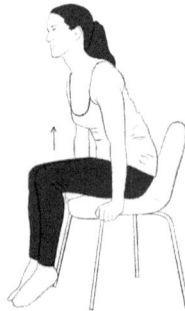

This movement builds strength in the muscles that support you when you're standing and sitting. It also improves your balance.

1. Begin by sitting up in your chair with your knees hip-width apart and your feet on the ground, toes pointing forward. Place your hands on the sides of your chair.
2. Bend forward as if you're going into a Seated Forward Fold, keeping your back and neck straight and in line.
3. Staying in this forward position, slowly lift up from your chair (about six inches) and then lower back down, returning to your seated position.
4. Repeat this pose eight times.

EAGLE ARMS

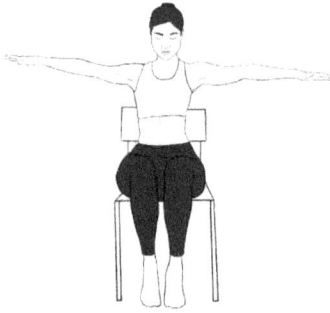

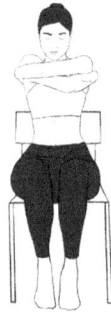

This posture helps to stabilize and flex your shoulder joints while relaxing your upper back and shoulders.

1. To begin, come to the Mountain pose.
2. As you inhale, extend your arms up and out to your sides.

3. As you exhale, bring your arms forward placing your right arm under your left arm and holding your shoulders with opposite hands, as if you're giving yourself a hug. If you have more flexibility in your shoulders, you can keep wrapping your arms until the palms of your hands are touching each other, instead of touching your shoulders.

4. Inhale and lift your arms a little higher. Exhale to release your arms back to your sides.

5. Repeat this movement on the opposite side with your left arm going under your right. Do this pose at least three times.

FULL BODY STRETCH WITH WEIGHTS

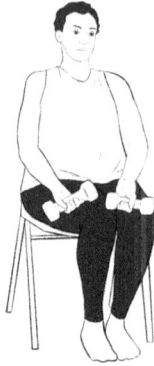

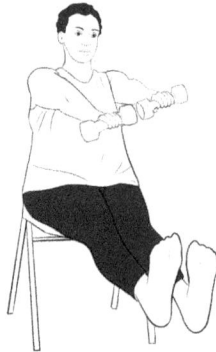

This pose not only strengthens all your muscles, but the addition of weights helps to tone those muscles.

1. Begin in Mountain pose, holding a two-pound weight in each hand, and rest your hands on your thighs.

2. As you breathe in, lift your arms and legs up at the same time. Try to keep your back straight. If you feel like you're slouching, lower your arms and legs a little until you feel like you can stay straight.

3. As you exhale, slowly lower your arms and legs back to your starting position.

4. Repeat this movement eight times. Once you're done, return to the Mountain pose and observe your breath. Notice how your body feels.

6

ADVANCED POSES

These poses require a bit more effort as well as strength and mobility. If you've been practicing for a while you can definitely try these. You can also combine or mix some of the beginner or intermediate poses with these for a slightly more intense practice.

SEATED CAT-COW

This pose helps to relieve tension in your back and shoulders while giving you a great stretch along your spine. It also helps to strengthen the muscles of the back.

1. Begin by sitting up tall in Mountain pose.

2. Inhale and slowly begin to arch your spine, rolling your shoulders back and down.
3. As you breathe out, round your spine, draw your belly in, and bring your chin to your chest.
4. Repeat these movements for five breaths.

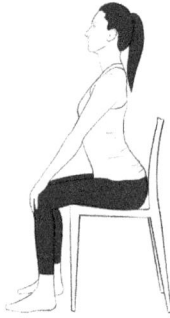

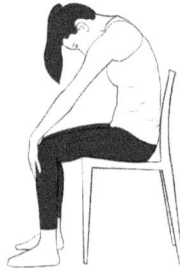

REVERSE ARM HOLD

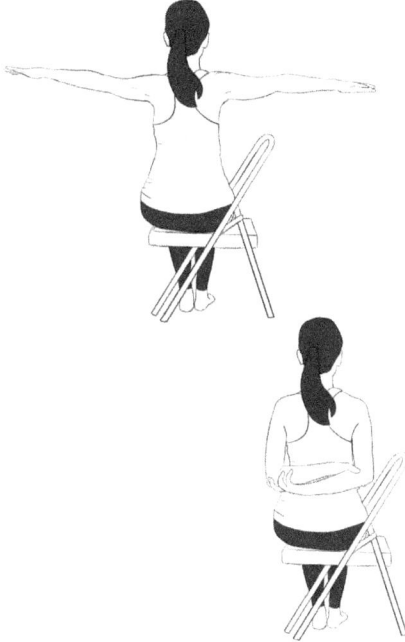

In addition to helping you relax, this pose helps to open up tight shoulders and stretches your chest, increasing mobility and flexibility in your shoulder joints.

1. Begin by sitting up straight with your knees hip-width apart.

2. As you inhale, lift both arms up and out to your sides with the palms facing down.

3. Exhale and gently swing both arms behind you and clasp your elbows with opposite arms. Take three slow breaths here, then release.

4. Repeat the movements, clasping the opposite way.

SEATED LOW LUNGE

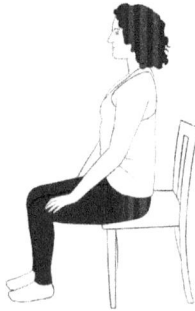

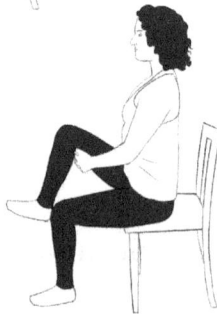

This pose can be restorative and is great for those who have hip pain or tightness in the hips. It strengthens the floor of the pelvis and helps to stabilize your hips.

1. Begin in Mountain pose.
2. Clasp your hands under your right thigh and on an inhale slowly raise your right knee towards your chest. Hold for one breath and release. If you find the pose difficult, sit all the way back in your chair and only lift the knee as far as feels comfortable.
3. Repeat the movement with the left leg. Try to do it at least eight times for each leg.

SEATED WARRIOR I

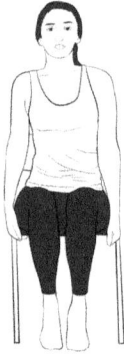

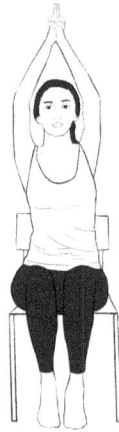

This pose improves circulation in your body and stretches the muscles in your arms.

1. Start in Mountain pose.
2. As you inhale, slowly lift your arms above your head. Interlace your fingers leaving the index

fingers free and pointing up. Take a moment to notice where your shoulders are. Try to relax them down and away from your ears.

3. Take five slow breaths, then release your hands.
4. Repeat this movement five times.

SEATED SIDE ANGLE

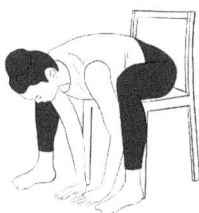

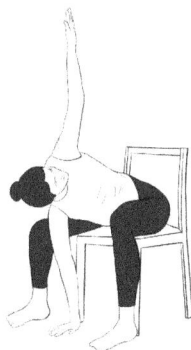

Seated Side Angle engages your core while stretching and strengthening your chest, shoulders, and lungs.

1. Come to a Seated Forward Fold but extend your arms down to the floor.
2. Place your left fingertips on the floor or a block.
3. As you inhale, open your chest and twist to your right lifting your right arm up toward the ceiling. You can look up at your right arm if it feels comfortable. Hold here for three breaths, then release back to your Seated Forward Fold.
4. Repeat with your right fingertips on the floor and your left arm extended.
5. Try to do this movement at least five times on each side.

SEATED PIGEON POSE

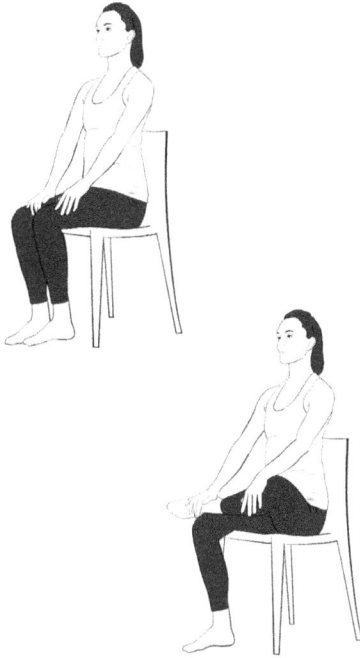

If you suffer from digestive issues this pose can help to alleviate some of the discomfort. It also stretches and strengthens your glutes and groin.

1. Come to sitting straight with your feet firmly planted on the floor, knees hip-distance apart and toes pointing forward.

2. Bring your right ankle up and place it on your left knee. Try not to let your left leg collapse inward.

3. Hold this pose for five breaths, then repeat with the other leg.

4. Do this at least three times for each leg.

FIVE-POINT STAR

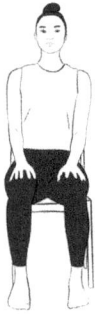

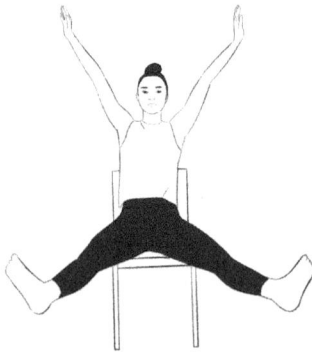

This pose is fantastic for your posture. It aligns, strengthens, and lengthens your spine. Not to mention, it's a great total body stretch.

1. Begin in Mountain pose.
2. On an inhale, extend your arms and legs out at the same time to create a star shape. If extending your arms and legs at the same time is difficult, do the arms first and then the legs. Remember, only go as far as feels right to you.
3. Exhale and release back to Mountain pose.
4. Complete this pose three times.

CHAIR CORPSE POSE

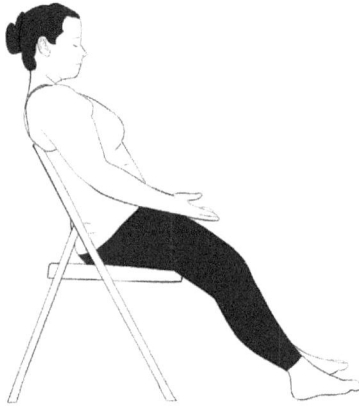

This is just about the best way to end your practice, refocus on yourself and notice your breath.

1. From your seated position, lean back in your chair, extend your legs out in front of you, and let your arms rest loose at your sides.
2. Close your eyes and simply observe your breath and the sensations. You can practice your meditation at this point if you would like.

CONCLUSION

Yoga is not only about caring for the physical body. It seeks to create harmony and balance between the mind, body, and spirit. You can practice yoga anywhere, at any time simply by taking a few moments to connect with your breath and notice how you're feeling.

Yoga can help to relax or calm you in stressful situations and it can make you stronger and more independent in your daily activities. Yoga is not just to be practiced on your chair but in your life.

The tools and poses that have been shared in this book are just stepping stones for you to lead a healthier, happier, calmer, and more independent life. As you begin or continue your yoga journey, try to remain consistent and persistent. Patience and steadiness are part of your yoga practice, so include them in your daily life. Above all else, enjoy it.

REFERENCES

Carraco, M. (2007, August 28). *A beginner's guide to meditation*. Yoga Journal. https://www.yogajournal.com/meditation/how-to-meditate/let-s-meditate/

Cherry, K. (2020, September 1). *What is meditation?* Verywell Mind. https://www.verywellmind.com/what-is-meditation-2795927

Cohut, M. (2017, August 27). *How yoga, meditation benefit the mind and body*. Www.medicalnewstoday.com. https://www.medicalnewstoday.com/articles/319116

Cronkleton, E. (2021, April 14). *Yoga for osteoporosis: 5 beneficial poses & how to do them*. Healthline. https://www.healthline.com/health/osteoporosis/yoga-for-osteoporosis#1

Ekhart, E. (2014, June 25). *The importance of breath in yoga*. Ekhart Yoga. https://www.ekhartyoga.com/articles/practice/the-importance-of-breath-in-yoga

Hastings, C. (2017, August 2). *Science shows yoga may protect your brain in old age.* World Economic Forum. https://www.weforum.org/agenda/2017/08/science-shows-yoga-may-protect-your-brain-in-old-age

Hullet, A. (2020, August 27). *Take a seat: 11 chair yoga poses to try.* Greatist. https://greatist.com/move/chair-yoga?c=643257173729#11-chair-yoga-poses-to-try

Lehmkuhl, L. (2020). *Chair yoga for seniors: Stretches and poses that you can do sitting down at home.* Skyhorse Publishing.

McGee, K. (2017, March 30). *Chair yoga meditation: Stillness as a complement to movement. Kristin McGee.* https://kristinmcgee.com/chair-yoga-meditation

Nichols, H. (2021, April 14). *Yoga: Methods, types, philosophy, and risks.* Www.medicalnewstoday.com. https://www.medicalnewstoday.com/articles/286745

Stelter, G. (2015, December 7). *Chair yoga for seniors: Seated poses.* Healthline. https://www.healthline.com/health/fitness-exercise/chair-yoga-for-seniors

Yoga Anytime. (2019, August 23). *Yoga breathing 101: Beginner tips and practices.* Yoga Anytime. https://www.

yogaanytime.com/blog/meditation/yoga-breathing-
101-beginner-tips-and-practices

www.ingramcontent.com/pod-product-compliance
Lightning Source LLC
Chambersburg PA
CBHW032154020426
42334CB00016B/1277